A New Look at ADHD
Inhibition, Time, and Self-Control

Video Manual

•◆•

Russell A. Barkley

THE GUILFORD PRESS
New York   London

BS

This manual is a companion to the videotape *A New Look at ADHD: Inhibition, Time, and Self-Control.*

2/27/07

Contents

•◆•

Preface   4

Introduction to ADHD   7

Why a New Theory of ADHD   12

Constructing the Theory of Self-Regulation and ADHD   14

Extending the Model of Self-Regulation to ADHD   28

Implications for Treating ADHD   31

References   37

Suggested Reading   38

Suggested Videos   39

Resources   39

About the Author   40

Preface

•◆•

This manual accompanies the videotape *A New Look at ADHD: Inhibition, Time, and Self-Control*. Both describe a totally new framework for understanding attention-deficit/hyperactivity disorder (ADHD) that I have devised in the hope of facilitating more effective interventions that will promise a brighter future for all children and adults who suffer from this widespread disorder. For 16 years I have been troubled by questions left unanswered by the long-held view that ADHD results largely from a deficit in attention. Stimulated by the seminal work of Dr. Jacob Bronowski (1977) conducted 25 years ago and buttressed by neuropsychological research in the past decade and a half, I have investigated the mechanisms behind ADHD and have concluded that ADHD is a deficit *not in attention but in behavioral inhibition*. The inability to delay action in response to an event leaves those who have ADHD with myriad cognitive deficits and, ultimately, poor self-control, a flawed sense of the future, and little grasp of themselves across time. What looks like inattention to the parents, teachers, and clinicians who have been observing these children results from an inability to regulate their behavior internally rather than remain governed, as very young infants are, by external stimuli.

The new theory presented in this manual and video offers a richer conceptualization of ADHD that not only explains the inattention and many of the other multiple cognitive deficiencies associated with the disorder (Barkley, 1997b, 1998), but also predicts additional impairments that merit scientific scrutiny. Ultimately, it provides far greater insight into the nature of ADHD and a deeper understanding of the approaches to treatment that will be needed to manage the symptoms of the disorder.

While parts of the model presented here have not been studied sufficiently to give them substantial support, mounting evidence

4

suggests that this or a very similar model will be required to account for what is known about the cognitive deficits found in ADHD. To unravel the complicated mystery of ADHD will require much more scientific study. For now, however, this theory advances our understanding by revealing, for example, why some treatments of the past and present may have been effective while others failed. It is my fond hope that this new view of ADHD will encourage others to build on this understanding to help those with ADHD look forward to more fruitful, successful lives.

The scientific basis for this model of self-regulation and the executive functions that permit it has been reviewed in detail elsewhere (Barkley, 1997b), along with the scientific evidence for its applicability to ADHD. I will only touch on a few highlights here. The bulk of this manual is devoted to explaining the key features of the new theory of ADHD, how this theory differs from the longstanding consensus view of the disorder, where it might lead in the development of future interventions, and what questions remain for us to explore. For more information, please refer to *ADHD and the Nature of Self-Control* (Barkley, 1997a) and to the other resources listed in "References" and "Suggested Reading."

This video and manual can be used to supplement materials for undergraduate or graduate courses in abnormal psychology, developmental psychopathology, general clinical psychology, psychiatry, or clinical social work. They can be used in parent training courses for families wishing to better understand and help manage their children who have ADHD. Or they can be integrated into group counseling of adults with ADHD, where they can be used by participants to help them learn more about their disorder. Of course, the video and manual can be used in the in-service training of mental health and special education professionals desiring to learn the latest view of ADHD and its implications for understanding, evaluating, and managing the disorder. (Additional manuals can be ordered separately from the publisher to serve as handouts for such workshops.)

My sincere appreciation goes to the individuals with ADHD who appear in this video. I salute their courage in sharing their views of this disorder with the general public. Thanks also go to my good friends and colleagues, Kevin Murphy, PhD, and Gwen Edwards, PhD, for agreeing to be interviewed for this project. Much gratitude is owed to Steve Lerner, PhD, psychologist and producer, for his collaboration on the video. As should be clear to anyone who views this video, his talents as a producer are exceptional. It was no easy feat bringing this theory to life in a visual medium and making it comprehensible to a general audience. I believe Steve has accomplished all this masterfully. I also want to thank Chris Benton and Anna Brackett, of The Guilford Press, for their skillful editing and production of this manual, and my good friends Robert Matloff and Seymour Weingarten at Guilford for their support of this project and their confidence that a video about a theory of ADHD would be of considerable benefit to those seeking a better understanding of this relatively common disorder. Finally, Steve and I thank the University of Massachusetts Medical School and the Fay School of Southborough, Massachusetts, for permitting us to use their facilities during the filming of this video.

RUSSELL A. BARKLEY
University of Massachusetts Medical School

Introduction to ADHD

•◆•

Children displaying the symptoms currently known as attention-deficit/hyperactivity disorder (ADHD)—inattention, poor impulse control, and hyperactivity or excessive motor movement (Barkley, 1998)—captured the attention of scientists as early as the beginning of the 20th century. Since 1902, when English physician George Still characterized a group of his patients as having a deficit in "volitional inhibition" or a "defect in moral control" (Barkley, 1997b), clinicians and researchers have been trying to understand this constellation of symptoms that makes it difficult for children to learn and socialize, to remember and plan, to behave the way "normal" children learn to behave over the first 18 years of their lives. Parents, teachers, and health care professionals have been vexed by the relative inability of these children to pay attention—to stick with their efforts toward completing tasks and activities, particularly those the child finds uninteresting—and to resist being drawn away by distractions. They have been frustrated by the fact that such children cannot seem to delay their initial dominant or reflexive response to an event long enough to "think better" before acting on impulse. And they have wrestled with the disruptiveness of children who fidget, cannot sit still, move around in ways unrelated to the task at hand, and generally behave or respond excessively, as if driven to move, squirm, manipulate, talk, run, or climb. Although neuropsychology and other fields of research have recently shed much light on the etiology of ADHD, we still have much to learn about the mechanisms behind these symptoms and why ADHD occurs in some children and not in others.

We do know that ADHD is a developmental disorder: the abilities to concentrate on tasks and avoid distractions, to "look before you leap," and to sit still in a classroom, for example, develop along a somewhat predictable course in normal children. In those with

ADHD, these abilities remain elusive well beyond the ages at which they usually appear. By 4 to 6 years of age, normal children are starting to become more compliant, inhibited, socialized, and willing to conform to situational norms and expectations. They are also able to attend to assigned activities for progressively longer periods of time, to resist distractions that interrupt those activities, and to restrain their initial urges to act on their impulses. Prior to the period 4–6, of course, most normal children can be quite active, inattentive, impulsive, and generally poorly self-controlled—especially if they are male. As a consequence, deficiencies in the rate of development of these powers of self-regulation often do not become evident until late preschool or early school age. Not surprisingly, it is often a child's teacher who first notices that a child has the symptoms of ADHD.

Self-regulation in normal individuals continues to develop well into the second and third decades of life. But those who are diagnosed with ADHD have up to an 80% chance of continuing to meet diagnostic criteria for the disorder (see American Psychiatric Association, 1994) into their adolescent years. In fact, the mental health profession now recognizes that adults can have this disorder, though until recently it was thought to be an affliction of childhood exclusively. Those diagnosed as children have up to a 70% chance of retaining the diagnosis into adulthood, and many of those who no longer meet the full clinical diagnostic criteria for ADHD continue to demonstrate poor self-regulation as adolescents or adults.

Socially cooperative animals that we are, the consequences of failure to develop self-control can be devastating. It is rare for a child or an adult with ADHD to experience no problems or impairments in functioning beyond the primary symptoms of ADHD. Across development, individuals diagnosed with ADHD are more likely than others to develop associated problems, or comorbid disorders. A pattern of irritable, defiant, stubborn, argumentative, and socially aggressive behavior known as "oppositional defiant disorder" may develop in as many as 40–67% of children with ADHD.* Of these, half or more may go on to develop "conduct disorder," a more serious pattern of behavior involving the violation of social rules and laws and the rights of others—in other words, 20–56% of all ADHD children may develop this additional disorder. These children and

---

*This manual reflects recent data not available at the time the video was shot.

teens are the most prone to delinquency, early substance experimentation and abuse, school failure, suspensions and expulsions, and later adult antisocial personality disorder (11–18%). Emotional problems are also more common in children with ADHD, with as many as 25% demonstrating one or more anxiety disorders and as many as 25–30% developing major depression. More recently it was discovered that children with ADHD may also be somewhat more likely to have manic depression, or bipolar disorder (1–6%), although the vast majority of children who have ADHD are not prone to this condition.

Besides these psychiatric risks, there are social ones as well. At least 50% of all children with ADHD will have serious interpersonal problems in their peer relationships; many will never have close friends as a result. But it is certainly in the educational setting where children with ADHD are most likely to have difficulties. As many as 90% of them are underperforming in schoolwork, usually involving underproductivity. Studies find that 25–50% or more also have a learning disability (LD), which saddles them with a second disorder that, while not directly due to their ADHD, surely interacts with it to further increase their risk for educational failure.

As adults, individuals with ADHD are more likely to have difficulties in their employment similar to the sorts of problems they demonstrated in school. They often do not work up to their potential, they require greater supervision and guidance than others, and they are less able to carry out independent projects. They also behave more impulsively, aggressively, and emotionally in the workplace. They will change jobs more often and are also more likely to be fired from their jobs than are other adults who do not have ADHD.

ADHD also affects other areas of daily life functioning in adulthood. These include motor vehicle driving (more accidents and speeding tickets), money management (poor budgeting, impulsive spending), sexual functioning (less use of birth control, greater risk for teen pregnancy and sexually transmitted diseases), and management of legal substances (greater predisposition to tobacco and alcohol use). Interpersonal problems with others are also evident in the majority of adults with ADHD.

As the video states, as many as 3 million American children and more than twice as many adults have ADHD today. Without appropriate intervention, a sizable segment of the U.S. population has dim prospects for a fulfilling life. This is why it is so important that we learn as much as possible about the nature and etiology of ADHD.

What Causes ADHD?

Research into the causes of ADHD has repeatedly identified neurology, heredity, and genetics as the most likely contributors to the disorder.

Neurology

Neuroimaging research (magnetic resonance images, or MRIs) has shown that children with ADHD have slightly smaller regions in the frontal part of the brain and in other structures interconnected to these regions (striatum, globus pallidus, cerebellum), particularly on the right side. Though the neuroimaging studies showed no brain damage in these areas, studies of cerebral blood flow have consistently shown decreased blood flow to the same regions. These regions seem to be less active than normal, giving rise to the hallmark symptoms of the disorder. A 1997 study strengthened the causal connection by finding a correlation between poor behavioral response inhibition and smaller size in these regions of the brain (Barkley, 1997b). Much is still unknown, however, about the neurological causes of ADHD. Researchers are now using advanced functional neuroimaging methods to study these brain regions and to try to link these findings to those on the genetics of the disorder.

Heredity and Genetics

A significant number of twin studies have shown that the expression and individual variation in the degree of ADHD in the population seems to be influenced largely by genetics. At least 80–90% of the variance in inattention, impulsiveness, and hyperactivity is the result of genetic effects. Studies of adopted children have confirmed the heritability of ADHD by showing that children usually resemble their biological parents in the symptoms of ADHD more than they resemble their adoptive parents. Research has also shown that siblings of children with ADHD have a 32% risk of having the disorder as well (as compared to the average risk of 3–5%), and that children of parents with ADHD have a 57% risk of having the disorder too (Barkley, 1997b).

ADHD is a complex disorder, and so it is highly likely that multiple genes play a role in creating the condition. Although no genes for ADHD have been reliably identified as yet, several candidate genes have been found to be associated to a greater than normal extent with ADHD. These findings prompt optimism that the genes for this disorder will be identified within the next decade, if not earlier.

It is important to note that ADHD has not been shown to result from chromosomal abnormalities (such as those in Down syndrome). Nor does it seem to be brought about the way genes cause hereditary diseases such as Tay–Sachs or cystic fibrosis. Instead, current speculation is that the genes responsible for the development of normal inhibition and self-regulation when they occur in the right combination occur in a different combination in ADHD, resulting in less-than-normal inhibition and self-control.

According to this theory, ADHD should not be considered a categorical disorder, pathology, or disease in most people having the disorder, but rather a cluster of symptoms that occur at one end of the continuum representing the varying ability of the population to sustain attention, resist distraction, inhibit behavior, and self-regulate. Those who fall closer to the norm may experience occasional problems with these abilities, but not to the extent that their major life activities are impaired. Those who fall closer to the low end of the continuum will suffer impairments severe enough to warrant diagnosis and treatment.

Injury

A small percentage of children do not inherit their ADHD but may develop it as a consequence of experiencing some insult to their brain, either during pregnancy or, to a lesser extent, during their childhood years. These constitute a minority of cases that are truly pathological in nature, given that the children acquired the disorder by some injurious process.

The Role of Environment

The twin studies and others have shown that ADHD is not caused by environmental factors, whether the parental management of the child, diet, the general rearing environment, or the child's home life. Social factors can, however, contribute to how successfully a child lives with ADHD and how high his or her risk is for developing oppositional defiant disorder, conduct disorder, anxiety, depression, and other disorders along with ADHD.

Why a New Theory of ADHD?

• ◆ •

We know much more about ADHD than we did 20 years ago, and many individuals have been helped by currently accepted interventions. What is the impetus for a new theory about the disorder? Why should we not just continue thinking of ADHD as comprised primarily of this triumvirate of problems with attention, inhibition, and motor activity?

As I have stated elsewhere (Barkley, 1997a, 1997b), a new paradigm for ADHD is needed for a number of reasons:

The current view of ADHD is atheoretical. The traditional consensus view of ADHD defines the disorder by *describing* its symptoms rather than by *explaining* them. As such, it is not a theory at all and is in fact something of a dead end. Any field of study must begin with a description of the phenomenon but then must go on to develop scientific theories about it. Without this maturation process, our understanding of the problem comes to a halt; our progress in treating it reaches a plateau. Theories are tools that can be put to work not only in helping us to better understand and explain the condition but also in making previously unexpected predictions about it that serve as the basis for new research initiatives. Theories guide the evaluation and treatment of any disorder more usefully than descriptions can.

The current view of ADHD does not attempt to link the understanding of the disorder with an understanding of normal child development in the areas of behavioral inhibition and self-control. That ADHD represents a developmental delay in response inhibition has been, since the early 1990s, a widely accepted premise among scientists. Yet characterizing ADHD as problems with attention, impulse control, and motor control says nothing about how the normal processes of development go awry to produce ADHD. For a theory of a disorder like ADHD to be persuasive, it must ultimately bridge the literature on that disorder with the larger literatures of developmental psychology and developmental neuropsychology as they pertain to normal development. As will be discussed later in this manual, the new theory posits that in ADHD the normal development of self-regulation and the executive functions related to it are being impaired by the core problem with behavioral inhibition (see Barkley, 1997b).

The theory described in this video and manual picks up where the clinical descriptions of and research findings on ADHD leave off. This theory describes the mental processes that lead from a delay in behavioral response inhibition in children with ADHD to the symptoms by which ADHD is currently viewed. It shows how behavioral inhibition is essential to the effective execution of four actions of self-regulation that serve to control behavior and make it more goal-directed, time-sensitive, and future-oriented (Barkley, 1997b). The theory breaks down a failure to inhibit behavior into specific underdeveloped functions and thus helps us understand *why* children with ADHD may not be able to complete their homework, keep quiet at the movies, or sit still in class. Perhaps most important, the theory includes a diversity of new and untested yet testable predictions about additional cognitive and behavioral deficits in ADHD deserving of further study but not addressed by the current paradigm. For instance, this theory predicts a deficit in working memory (remembering so as to do something later) in those with ADHD. It also predicts a disturbance of their sense of time, among other previously unconsidered deficits.

The current view treats the subtypes of ADHD as sharing qualitatively identical deficits in attention, and differing only in the presence or absence of hyperactive–impulsive symptoms. It is doubtful that the problems with "inattention" associated with hyperactive–impulsive behavior (hyperactive type and combined type of ADHD) lie in the realm of attention. More likely, they are the province of inhibition and self-regulation. However, those problems seen in the predominantly inattentive type do appear to be related to attention, if current research findings on this subtype continue to support some initial findings on the matter.

A good theory of ADHD will explain why such qualitative distinctions exist among these subtypes and may even show that the inattentive type is really a separate disorder from ADHD when it is defined properly.

The current view fails to explain many of the specific findings about children with ADHD. As I have discussed elsewhere (Barkley, 1995, 1997b), research and clinical observation have produced a collection of "orphan" findings that have no "parent" theory to account for them:

- How does impulsivity, hyperactivity, or inattentiveness explain the fact that Johnny lets whatever is at hand, rather than anything he could know about the future, govern his behavior?
- What does the triumvirate of problems have to do with the

fact that 9-year-old Jane uses self-talk that resembles that of her 6-year-old sister in sophistication?

- Why do children with ADHD have trouble doing math in their heads when they exhibit no deficiency in math comprehension?
- Why do children with ADHD have trouble organizing themselves and contributing to cooperative group projects in school?
- Why does 12-year-old Rosa repeatedly get into trouble for "borrowing" classmates' belongings and "forgetting" to return them, when 8-year-old Misha can predict the consequences every time?
- If children with ADHD have a deficit in attention—in accurately perceiving incoming stimuli, as the video states—why are they able to play video games or watch television for hours on end?
- Why do children with ADHD improve their performance on lab tasks when an adult simply sits in the room with them?
- Why can't we predict how children with ADHD will perform and how well they will produce at different points in their development?

Constructing the Theory of Self-Regulation and ADHD

•◆•

The new theory of ADHD begins to explain the phenomena listed above or at least points us in the right direction for further research. As stated earlier, a delay in the development of inhibition in behavior is widely accepted as the underlying cause of all three of the hallmark symptoms of ADHD. But how does this delay work exactly?

My investigation into this process began with Dr. Bronowski's (1977) theory that being able to delay our response to any event allows us to separate our emotional reaction from objective information, develop a sense of past and future, talk to ourselves to control our behavior, and break up incoming data to recombine it into new responses. Without the brief delay that makes these functions possible, we cannot develop self-control. Because of their importance, these functions are called *executive functions*; they are the means by which we control our behavior internally rather than leaving it to the vagaries of the immediate environment. The model that I have constructed from this foundation ultimately has led me to believe that the brain's so-called central executive—the final arbiter in the mind's selection of goals and the data and plans to achieve them—is time and, with it, our sense of the future.

The Model

Self-regulation, or self-control, has a purpose critical to self-preservation: the anticipation of changes in the environment so as to maximize long-term benefits to the individual. The model of self-regulation on which this new theory of ADHD is based is a hybrid derived from several earlier models (see Barkley, 1997a, 1997b). It has three components:

1. Behavioral inhibition.
2. Executive functions.
3. Motor control system.

Self-regulation begins with behavioral inhibition. Behavioral inhibition, or the delay in response to an event, permits the brain's executive functions to occur. In fact, behavioral inhibition supports the occurrence of the executive functions and protects them from interference. These functions direct and guide behavior through the final component of the model, the motor control system. Once a goal-directed behavior has been chosen through the executive functions and is put into action by the motor control system, behavioral inhibition protects those behaviors from being disrupted by distracting events as necessary.

Behavioral Inhibition:
The Foundation of Self-Control

Behavioral inhibition is, of course, the ability to delay a response. But its ramifications are much broader. This ability makes it possible to stop an ongoing response that is proving ineffective and to protect the mental effort taking place during this delay from disruption by competing events and responses (also called *interference control*).

Without inhibition, self-control is difficult, if not impossible.

Self-control allows us to modify our behavior to change a delayed or future consequence associated with a particular event. This modification begins when we inhibit the initial, or prepotent, response or interrupt an ongoing response to an event. This delay gives us the time needed to engage in the four types of self-directed actions, or executive functions, included in the model presented here. That is, inhibition is necessary for this entire process to take place because it keeps the initial urge to act on impulse at bay while we think over the situation at hand and decide what to do. As shown in Figure 1,

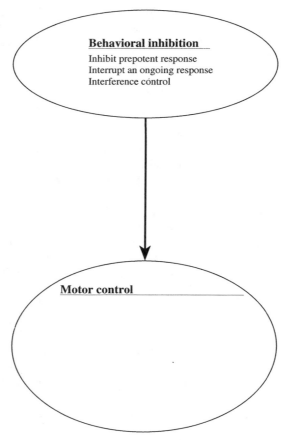

FIGURE 1. The influence of the behavioral inhibition system on the motor control system.

behavioral inhibition exerts a direct influence over the behavioral programming and motor control system of the brain.

The Executive Functions

Once the initial urge to respond is inhibited, the executive system can be engaged to determine the most appropriate response to the situation. As shown in Figure 2, this executive system is made up of four executive functions, each a general type of self-directed behavior used to exercise self-control.

As mentioned earlier, the executive functions internalize behavior for the purpose of anticipating change in the environment. That change represents essentially the concept of time (a sequence of events). And so the internalization of behavior results in the internalization of a sense of time. That sense of time and the future allow us to organize our behavior in anticipation of change. Those who

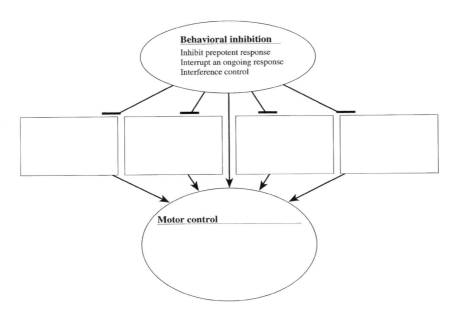

FIGURE 2. The relationship of the behavioral inhibition system to four executive functions (boxes) and their relationship to the motor control system.

develop behavioral inhibition normally should then have the capacity to become goal-directed, purposive, and intentional in their actions. Like language development, this developmental process of internalizing our self-directed behavior and the sense of time it provides is universal to all normal human beings. It is an instinct, not merely a product of cultural training.

While I believe that each of these executive functions is capable of being separated from the others, all of them are interactive and interreliant in their naturally occurring state. This is a critical point. *It is the action of these functions in concert, like an orchestra playing a symphony, that permits and produces normal human self-regulation.* Deficits in any particular executive function will produce a relatively distinct impairment in self-regulation, different from the impairment in self-control produced by deficits in the other functions.

The first executive function is *nonverbal working memory,* essentially the ability to engage in sensing to oneself. The most important senses to humans are vision and then hearing, and so this function is largely comprised of seeing to ourselves (visual imagery) and hearing to ourselves. But this executive ability also involves the other senses.

The second executive function has been called *verbal working memory* by some researchers. It is essentially the use of self-speech (the mind's voice).

The third function is the *internalization or self-regulation of emotion.* Along with it comes also the internalization of motivation. That is because our emotions are based on our sense of the consequences that may occur. And so the emotional centers of the brain provide the strong signals we feel to act.

The fourth and final executive function I call *reconstitution.* It is the process of analysis and synthesis that leads to creative problem solving and arises, I believe, from the internalization of play.

Behavioral inhibition and at least three of these executive functions appear to be mediated by separate but surely interactive regions of the prefrontal lobes (see Barkley, 1997b). Behavioral inhibition and its component processes seem to be localized to the orbital–frontal regions and its interconnections to the striatum. Accumulating evidence suggests that persistent inhibition or resistance to distraction (interference control) may be somewhat more lateralized to the right anterior prefrontal region, but the capacity to inhibit prepotent responses so as to delay the decision to respond seems well situated in the orbito–prefrontal region. Working memory (both verbal and nonverbal) seems to be associated with the dorsolateral or outside regions of the prefrontal cortex. And the regulation of affect–motivation–arousal has been attributed to the ventral–medial regions located on the walls in the central valley between the two hemispheres of the prefrontal lobes.

Undoubtedly, these executive functions and the future-directed forms of behavior they permit do not all arise suddenly or simultaneously in human development. There are likely to be phases or stages to their development, arising as they probably do in some staggered sequence during maturation. I have conjectured that behavioral inhibition arises first and quite likely just ahead of or in parallel with the nonverbal working memory functions. This is followed in all likelihood by the internalization of affect and motivation. Close on its heels comes the progressive internalization of speech. Finally, there is the internalization of play, or the creative problem-solving component of the model (reconstitution). Far more research will be needed to indicate whether this sequence is accurate. Here I wish to emphasize only that the executive functions seem to develop in stages.

Interestingly, these executive functions generally are publicly observable in a child's early development—and may also have been so early in human evolution—but become progressively more private or covert in form. The development of internalized, self-directed speech is an example. Children progress from simply talking to others to talking out loud to themselves to talking to themselves in their heads. This final covert stage of self-speech is verbal thought, but it is still technically just speech to the self. Over development, then, public behavior directed toward others gives rise to behavior directed at the self, which in turn gives rise to a more private, unobservable form of self-directed behavior: thinking.

Nonverbal Working Memory

Nonverbal working memory, shown in Figure 3, is the capacity to hold information in the mind so it can be used to control a subsequent response. It represents the covert sensing to oneself of an event, a response, and an outcome. While it includes all forms of sensory–motor behavior, the two that are particularly important to human self-regulation are covert visual imagery (seeing to oneself) and covert audition (hearing to oneself). Through this executive function we literally "see" the future in our mind's eye and use this image to direct and guide our behavior toward the goal we imagine.

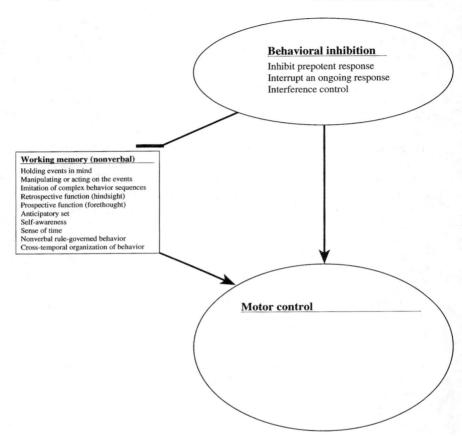

FIGURE 3. The functions of the nonverbal working memory system and its relationship to the behavioral inhibition and motor control systems.

This ability to revisualize the past is called *hindsight* or, as in the video, *retrospection.* Through this facility we bring our pertinent past history forward into the moment to inform our decisions about what to do next. Over development, each of us builds up a progressively larger archive of past experiences that can be reactivated in this way.

A parallel process that arises out of hindsight is called *fore-thought* or, as in the video, *foresight,* or *prospection.* The sense of past brings with it a sense of what was done before and what might be done next. In this way, hindsight creates forethought. The recall of the past thus permits anticipation of a future and primes our motor responses, referred to as *anticipatory set.*

Seeing our past to ourselves so as to anticipate and prepare for our future creates in all of us a sense of self-awareness. But it is self-awareness across time. Working memory therefore also appears to provide the basis for the human sense of time.

One facility that people with ADHD seem to lack and that working memory seems to underlay is the development of a preference for deferred gratification. In a way, the development of hindsight and forethought creates a window on time (past, present, future) of which the individual is aware. The temporal opening of that window probably increases across development, at least up to age 30 years. This might suggest that across child and adolescent development, the individual comes to organize and direct behavior toward events that lie increasingly distant in the future. By adulthood (ages 20–81), behavior is being organized to deal with events of the near future (8–12 weeks ahead) most often, but can be extended to events later in time if the consequences associated with those events are particularly salient. One means, then, of judging the maturity of a person's time horizon at differing ages is to examine the average period before an event when the person typically begins to make preparations for that event.

Another powerful tool that working memory affords us is the ability to imitate the complex sequences of behavior demonstrated by others. This occurs because we can review the behavior of another in our mind's eye and so use this image as the template to build our copy of that behavior. Through such imitation we learn new behaviors, manufacture and use tools, and share in a common culture.

It is not difficult to imagine that those with ADHD, if they are not afforded the delay in response that behavioral inhibition permits, may not learn from their own mistakes, from the example of others, or from the culture at large.

Verbal Working Memory

Verbal working memory (see Figure 4), or the internalization of speech, can be thought of as the mind's voice. This is the facility by which we label, describe, and verbally contemplate the nature of an event or situation. We also use verbal working memory to ask ourselves questions and give ourselves instructions. Most children develop the ability to internalize their speech by age 12. Before that,

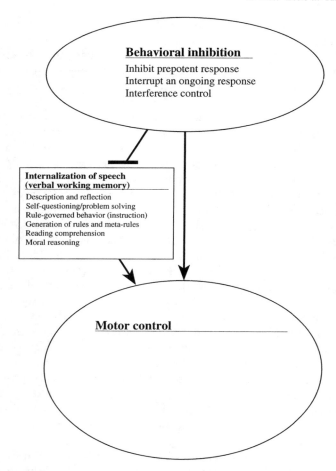

FIGURE 4. The functions of the verbal working memory system and its relationship to the behavioral inhibition and motor control systems.

they direct their speech outward at others and then speak aloud to themselves. When verbal and nonverbal working memory interact, they allow us to plan, solve problems, and strategize. They may also contribute to mental abilities such as reading comprehension and moral reasoning. An important function of verbal working memory is the formulation of rules and, eventually, rules about rules (*meta-rules*), generated into a hierarchically arranged system.

A person who has ADHD may act impulsively because she is

not privy to the mental talk that would tell her what an event means and what the rules for that situation are.

Self-Regulation of Emotion

In addition to sensing to ourselves and speaking to ourselves, we have the capacity to emote, or to motivate ourselves, as shown in Figure 5. This executive function provides the drive to persist toward future goals in the absence of external rewards.

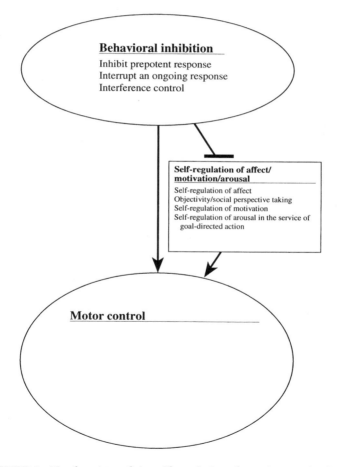

FIGURE 5. The functions of the self-regulation of emotion, motivation, and arousal system to the behavioral inhibition and motor control systems.

Damasio (1994, 1995) noted that visual imagery and covert self-speech produce not only private images and verbalizations but also the emotional charges associated with them, which he called *somatic markers*. Our private, mental deliberations concerning the decision to respond will not only result in a modification of what we choose to do but also influence the eventual emotional charge associated with that response. Such use of private action to countermand or counterbalance the initial emotional charge of external events contributes to the development of *emotional self-control*. For example, rather than shout when bruised, a child may stifle a loud "Ow!" by remembering that it will not hurt for long, by knowing that his peers do not behave that way in reaction to a minor bump, and by telling himself to bite his lip to avoid crying.

Besides permitting us to control our expression of emotion, this executive function arouses and motivates us to pursue and persist with our goals. By visualizing our goals and their outcomes, we can, to a certain degree, feel the emotions associated with those outcomes, and this serves to motivate us to persist toward those goals. The array of human emotions can be reduced to a two-dimensional grid of which one dimension is *motivation* (reinforcement and punishment) and the other *arousal*. Emotions are the result of continual appraisals of the external world; they inform us about the significance of events to our own concerns and thus motivate action. When we visualize outcomes, we can then also appraise them in our mind. And this helps us choose which ones to pursue. But our use of such private emotions can also be reinforced by the consequences of a certain level of arousal they create in us. If getting "fired up" by visualizing success pushes an athlete toward the finish line faster, the athlete will learn to self-induce the emotional state necessary to win the next race.

The persistence, willpower, determination, tenacity, and perseverance mentioned in the video are all products of this executive function. Impairment of this function may explain the so-called inattention or inability to persist toward a goal observed in those with ADHD.

Reconstitution

Shown in Figure 6, this executive function enables us to pull apart the behavior patterns we observe and put them back together into new responses. For this reason it is often called "reconstitution," but it may be more clearly understood as creative problem solving.

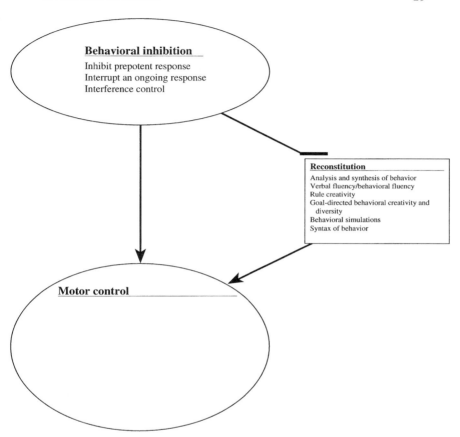

FIGURE 6. The functions of the reconstitution system and its relationship to the behavioral inhibition and motor control systems.

We use analysis and synthesis, the components of creative problem solving, every day. Human speech is one example: when we are asked a question, we must rapidly combine various words to create sentences that convey ideas to others. But we also use it in nonverbal behavior. Consider the ability to play the piano, which involves the rapid assembling of fine motor gestures by an accomplished pianist into extraordinarily complex sequences of the movements of digits on both hands simultaneously—a perfect example of analysis and synthesis, or taking apart and understanding components and then putting them back together. The marvel that results—and other forms of complex human motor responses and their reconstitution, such as ballet, gymnastics, drawing, handwriting, and architecture—cannot be matched by other animal species. Unlike other animals, we have a substantial power to create new behavior. Indeed, some would say our capacity to learn and create is infinite.

For those with ADHD, lacking this capacity robs them of the opportunity to mentally construct and test simulations of behaviors and thus avoid the unforeseen consequences that follow when they act on the first idea formulated.

Motor Control System

The motor control system is, in essence, the endpoint of the process of self-directed actions. Behavioral inhibition and the four other executive functions it supports take control of the motor system, wresting it from complete domination by the immediate environment. I call this component of the model *motor control/fluency/syntax* to emphasize the idea that the executive functions do not simply control and manage the motor system but must actually use a set of rules for assembling a behavioral sequence into complex new behavior, known as a *syntax*.

Figure 7 illustrates the completed model. How does it manifest in the behavior of a person who has developed normally? First, behavior that is unrelated to the goal becomes minimized or even suppressed during task completion or goal-directed action. Because of the power to generate motivation internally, the person can sustain behavior toward its intended destination. This creates *goal-directed persistence*—a persistence that is characterized by willpower, self-discipline, determination, single-mindedness of purpose, and a drivenness or intentional quality.

Throughout the execution of goal-directed behaviors, working memory permits the feedback from the last response(s) to be held in mind so as to feed forward in modifying subsequent responding. This creates *a sensitivity to errors*. Just as important, when interruptions in a chain of goal-directed behaviors occur, the individual is able to *disengage, respond to the interruption, and then reengage the original goal-directed sequence*. That is so because the plan for that goal-directed activity has been held in mind despite interruption.

As we shall see, the sequence is much different for those with ADHD.

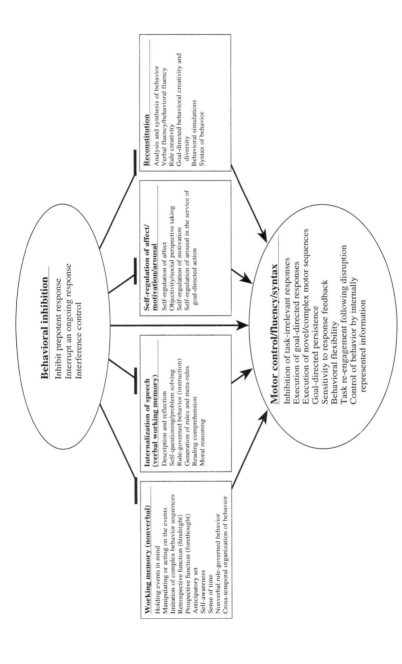

FIGURE 7. The complete hybrid model of executive functions (boxes) and the relationship of these four functions to the behavioral inhibition and motor control systems.

Behavioral inhibition
Inhibit prepotent response
Interrupt an ongoing response
Interference control

Working memory (nonverbal)
Holding events in mind
Manipulating or acting on the events
Imitation of complex behavior sequences
Retrospective function (hindsight)
Prospective function (forethought)
Anticipatory set
Self-awareness
Sense of time
Nonverbal rule-governed behavior
Cross-temporal organization of behavior

Internalization of speech (verbal working memory)
Description and reflection
Self-questioning/problem solving
Rule-governed behavior (instruction)
Generation of rules and meta-rules
Reading comprehension
Moral reasoning

Self-regulation of affect/ motivation/arousal
Self-regulation of affect
Objectivity/social perspective taking
Self-regulation of motivation
Self-regulation of arousal in the service of goal-directed action

Reconstitution
Analysis and synthesis of behavior
Verbal fluency/behavioral fluency
Rule creativity
Goal-directed behavioral creativity and diversity
Behavioral simulations
Syntax of behavior

Motor control/fluency/syntax
Inhibition of task-irrelevant responses
Execution of goal-directed responses
Execution of novel/complex motor sequences
Goal-directed persistence
Sensitivity to response feedback
Behavioral flexibility
Task re-engagement following disruption
Control of behavior by internally represented information

27

Extending the Model of Self-Regulation to ADHD

•◆•

The inhibitory deficit that characterizes ADHD disrupts the control of motor behavior by the executive system. In short, ADHD delays the development of the capacity to internalize behavior via the executive functions and thereby delays the self-regulation they afford to the individual.

Given all this, those with ADHD could be said to have impairments in all the executive functions and their subfunctions listed in Figure 7. Consequently, they would manifest difficulties in the motor control component of that model as well. This means that ADHD is not just a deficit in behavioral inhibition but also a deficit in executive functioning and self-regulation. This deficit results in a renegade motor control system that is not under the same degree of control by internally represented information, time, and the future as would be evident in the normal peer group of the person who has ADHD (see Figure 8).

The implications of this new theoretical model for understanding, diagnosing, assessing, and treating ADHD are numerous and far-reaching (see Barkley, 1997b). Two are particularly important to understanding how this theory changes our perceptions of ADHD and the possible avenues for intervention:

ADHD as a Disorder of Performance, Not of Skill

The totality of the deficits associated with ADHD serve to cleave thought from action, knowledge from performance, past and future from the moment, and the dimension of time from the rest of the three-dimensional world more generally. *This means that ADHD is not a disorder of knowing what to do but of doing what one knows.* ADHD is a disorder of applied intelligence; its deficits partially dissociate the crystallized intelligence of prior knowledge from its application in the day-to-day stream of adaptive functioning. ADHD, then, is a disorder of performance more than a disorder of skill, a disability more in the *when* and *where* and less in the *how* or *what* of behavior.

Those with ADHD often know what they should do or should have done before. They have the necessary skills to read a book, complete a math problem, listen to a lesson in school. But this provides little consolation to them, little influence over their behavior, and

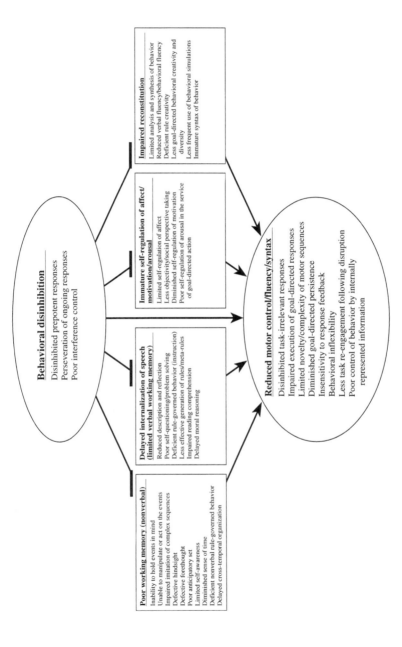

FIGURE 8. The hybrid model of executive functions (Figure 7) revised to show the numerous cognitive deficits predicted to be associated with deficits in behavioral inhibition of ADHD.

often much irritation to others. Because they respond on impulse, those with ADHD act as if they do not have such knowledge and skill when they are actually behaving at particular moments.

When others readily foresee events that lie ahead in the distant future, they initiate various planning and anticipatory actions. Those with ADHD do so much closer to the time of the event—if at all. This is a recipe for a life of chaos and crisis, with everything that needs to be done being left to the last minute. Individuals with ADHD squander their energies dealing with emergencies or urgencies at the eleventh hour when a few moments' forethought and planning could have eased the burden and likely headed off the crisis.

This new theory encourages an important shift in attitudes concerning ADHD. Understanding the disorder as more than a checklist of observable difficulties, as the video describes the traditional view, empowers both caregivers and those with ADHD to deal productively with the challenges they face. By confirming the neurological and genetic basis of the disorder, the new theory offsets societal tendencies to blame the patient—or for the patients to blame themselves—for their predicament.

Time as the Ultimate Disability

Understanding time and how we organize our own behavior within it and toward it is a major key to the mystery of understanding ADHD supplied by this new theory. I now believe that the *awareness of themselves across time is the ultimate yet nearly invisible disability afflicting those with ADHD.* When we view ADHD in this way, we undergo another shift in attitude toward the disorder.

For those who cannot see spatial distances very well, the solution is corrective lenses. For those who neglect to respond to events at visuo–spatial distances as a consequence of brain injury, the prescription is cognitive rehabilitation. But what are the solutions for those with a myopia or blindness to time? How can we help those who have a "temporal neglect syndrome"—a neglect of distances that lie ahead in time? And how can those individuals be expected to benefit from any corrective or rehabilitative treatments when the very cognitive mechanisms that subserve the use of these treatments—the self-regulatory or executive functions—are precisely where the damage caused by ADHD lies?

Teaching time awareness and time management to those who cannot *perform* time awareness or time management, no matter how much they may *know* about time awareness and time management, is not going to prove especially fruitful. Given the disability in performing within time, it would not be surprising to find that the person with ADHD may not show up on time or at all for the appointments for such rehabilitation most of the time.

Implications for Treating ADHD

• ◆ •

For those living with, teaching, and treating children and adults with ADHD, the knowledge that these individuals are not lacking intelligence but are lacking a sense of time obviously can revolutionize methods of interacting. With continuing research, I hope it will also continue to produce effective intervention techniques.

Treating at the Point of Performance

An important implication of this theory is that *the most useful treatments will be those that are in place in the natural settings where the desired behavior is to occur.* This setting is called the "point of performance," and it seems to be a key concept in the management of those with ADHD (Ingersoll & Goldstein, 1993). The farther away in space and time that any intervention takes place from this critical point of performance, the less effective it should be. This immediately suggests that clinic-delivered treatments, such as play therapy, counseling of the child, neurofeedback, and other such therapies are not likely to produce clinically significant improvement in ADHD, if any at all. Instead, the most effective treatments will be programs such as behavior modification that restructure the natural setting to encourage a change in the desired behavior. The goal is not to teach anything new but *to maintain that desired behavior over time.*

Treating Symptomatically

Treatments that alter the natural environment to increase desired behavior at critical points of performance will result in changes in that behavior and its maintenance over time *only insofar as the treatments are maintained* in those places over time. If the treatments are removed, most or all gains will be lost and the individual will return to pretreatment levels of symptoms. Behavioral treatments and other such methods of management applied at the point of performance do not alter the underlying neuropsychological and largely genetic deficits in behavioral inhibition. They only provide immediate relief from them by reducing or restructuring those environmental factors that appear to handicap the performance of the individual with ADHD in that setting. Such treatments, even when in place, also should not be expected to produce generalization of treatment effects to other settings where no such treatments are in place.

Thus treatment of the individual with ADHD is not so much a cure that eliminates the underlying cause of the disorder as a means of providing temporary, point-of-performance improvement in the symptoms. Such treatment may reduce the future risks that are secondary consequences of having unmanaged ADHD, but probably only if these short-term treatments are sustained over the long term. Nevertheless, the reduction of immediate distress and improvement in immediate success is a legitimate treatment outcome for improving the immediate quality of life for the individual with ADHD.

Treating Inhibition Deficits with Stimulant Medications

This understanding of how treatment may work suggests a more specific implication for the management of ADHD: only a treatment that can result in improvement or normalization of the underlying neuropsychological deficit in behavioral inhibition is likely to result in an improvement or normalization of the self-control that people with ADHD lack. To date, the only treatment that has any hope of achieving this end is stimulant medication or other psychopharmacological agents that temporarily improve or normalize the neural substrates in the prefrontal regions that likely underlie this disorder. The benefit of such medications accrues only while the medication remains within the brain.

Research shows that clinical improvement in behavior occurs in as many as 75–92% of those with the hyperactive–impulsive form of ADHD and results in normalization of behavior in approximately 50–60% of these cases, on average (Werry & Aman, 1998). Since it is the only treatment to date known to produce such improvement/ normalization rates, stimulant medication seems to be the best treatment approach for the management of ADHD currently available.

Society may view medication treatment of children with ADHD as anathema largely due to a misunderstanding of both the nature of ADHD specifically and the nature of self-control more generally. Many in society wrongly believe the causes of both ADHD and poor self-control to be chiefly social, particularly improper child rearing. Evidence of ADHD's genetic basis indicates that using stimulant medication to help temporarily improve or alleviate the underlying neuropsychological dysfunction therefore is a commendable, ethically and professionally responsible, and humane way of proceeding with treatment for those with ADHD.

Externalizing What Is Missing Internally

If ADHD results in an undercontrol of behavior by internalized, self-directed executive functions, then treatment should involve externalizing those functions as much as possible.

Externalizing Information

In ADHD, if the information that is supposed to be generated by the executive functions is being generated at all, it appears to be extraordinarily weak in controlling and sustaining behavior toward the future. Rather than being directed by verbal and nonverbal working memory, behavior remains largely under the control of the salient aspects of the immediate context.

The solution to this problem is not to carp at those with ADHD to simply try harder or to admonish them to remember what they are supposed to be working on or toward. It is instead to take charge of the immediate context and fill it with physically represented forms of information that are comparable to those internal counterparts that are proving so ineffective. In a sense, clinicians treating those with ADHD must "beat the environment at its own game." They must put into the immediate context the sorts of cues, prompts, physical reminders, and other captivating information that will guide behavior toward the intended goal. Sources of high-appealing distracters that may subvert, pervert, or disrupt task-directed behavior should be minimized where possible. In their place should be forms of stimuli and information that are just as salient and appealing yet are directly associated with or an inherent part of the task that is to be accomplished.

If the rules that are understood to be operative during classroom individual deskwork, for instance, do not seem to be controlling the behavior of a child with ADHD, posting signs about the classroom that are related to these rules or creating a poster displayed at the front of the class or typed on a card taped to the child's desk can externally remind the child of these rules. Having the child verbally self-state these rules out loud before and during these individual work performances may also be helpful. Tape-recording these reminders onto a cassette tape that the child listens to through an earphone while working would be another means of externalizing the rules. My textbook (Barkley, 1998) articulates the details of the many other treatments that could be designed from this model.

Externalizing a Sense of Time

Chief among these internally represented forms of information that need to be either externalized or removed entirely from the task are those related to time. Time and the future are the enemies of people with ADHD when it comes to task accomplishment or performance toward a goal. An obvious solution, then, is to reduce or eliminate the temporal elements of a task by making its elements more contiguous.

Take the example of a book report assigned today but due in 2 weeks, to be graded at least a week later, before being returned to the student. There is a 2-week gap between the event (assignment) and response (report) in this contingency, as well as a 1-week gap between the response and its consequence (the grade). Moreover, the reward for completing the task is abstract and thus a rather weak source of motivation for someone with ADHD. To reduce the detrimental impact of the temporal gaps in this project, the task should be structured as follows for the child with ADHD:

1. Read five pages *right now* from your book.
2. Then write two or three sentences for me *right now* based on what you have read.
3. When you have done that, I will give you five tokens (or some other immediate privilege) that you have earned for following this instruction.

This is a way of bridging time by taking small steps toward the longer term goal or target, a seemingly simplistic concept that is critical to developing effective management programs for those with ADHD.

When temporal parameters cannot be eliminated, the sense of time itself, or its passage, needs to be externalized to compensate for a distorted internal, cognitive clock. For instance, instead of telling a child with ADHD that he has 30 minutes to get a chore done, write that number on the card explaining the rules for the task and also place a spring-loaded kitchen timer set to 30 minutes where the child can see it while performing the task.

Externalizing Sources of Motivation and Drive

A major caveat must be added to all of these implications for externalizing forms of internally represented information: externalizing internalized forms of information is likely to prove only partially successful, and even then only temporarily. Internal sources of motivation must be augmented with more powerful external forms as well. Externalizing information without externalizing motivation is a sure recipe for ineffective treatment. Complaining to individuals with ADHD about their lack of motivation (laziness), drive, willpower, or self-discipline will not suffice. Nor will pulling back from assisting them so as to let the natural consequences occur, as if this will teach them a lesson that will correct their behavior. Instead, try using a token system, one of the best means for creating artificial reward programs for children 5 years of age and older. Plastic poker chips can be given throughout the task and at its end, as suggested earlier in the book report example. These chips can be exchanged for other, more salient privileges, rewards, or treats that the child with ADHD may desire. This concept applies as much to mild punishments for inappropriate behavior or poor work performance as it does to rewards.

As I have noted earlier, such artificial sources of motivation must be maintained over long periods of time, or the gains in performance they initially induce will not be sustained. However, because those with ADHD merely lag behind their normal peers in this capacity, children with ADHD can usually be weaned from reliance on external sources of motivation as they mature and develop the capacity for self-motivation. At any particular age, though, children with ADHD will still need these external sources of motivation more than normal individuals of the same age.

Addressing Deficits in Reconstitution

How to deal with the problem of reconstitution predicted to be defi-
cient in those with ADHD seems to me more difficult to address
than the deficits in the other executive functions. If more were
known about the process of analysis/synthesis and the behavioral creativity it gives rise to, ways of externalizing this process might be
more evident.

Perhaps placing the parts of an assigned problem on some externally represented material would help, along with prompting and
guidance on how to take apart and move about these forms of information so as to recombine them into more useful forms. Adults seem
to do this when struggling with a difficult problem; they make their
previous internal forms of problem-solving behavior external. For
instance, we see this happen when people talk to themselves out
loud while solving a difficult puzzle or acquiring a complex proce-
dure. They begin to doodle on a pad, and play with certain designs,
free-associate publicly to the topic of the problem under discussion,
or even reduce a number of words to slips of paper or pieces of mag-
nets and then randomly reshuffle them to create new arrangements.
(The game Magnetic Poetry does this with words on small magnetic
strips; Boggle, Scrabble, and anagrams achieve the same thing with
letters.)

If the task or problem is a verbal one, then a word-processing
program on a personal computer might prove useful. Having the
individual with ADHD just type as many pieces of information as
possible into the word-processing file would be the first step, ignor-
ing for the moment organization, grammar, and other issues. Once
the information is gotten down in some physical form, the person
can edit, move, and otherwise rearrange and sculpt this information
into a more finely honed document.

Managing ADHD as a Chronic Disability

All of the foregoing leads to a much more general implication of this
model of ADHD: the approach taken to its management must be
the same as is taken in the management of other chronic medical or
psychiatric disabilities. I have frequently used diabetes as an analo-
gous condition in trying to assist parents and other professionals in
grasping this point. At the time of diagnosis, it is realized that no

cure for the condition currently exists. Still, there are multiple means of providing symptomatic relief from the deleterious effects of the condition, some of which include taking daily doses of medication and others of which involve changing settings, tasks, and lifestyles. A treatment package of these means is designed and brought to bear on the condition immediately following diagnosis. This package must be maintained over long periods of time so as to maintain the symptomatic relief initially achieved by the treatments. It is hoped that the treatment package, so maintained, will reduce or eliminate the secondary consequences of leaving the condition unmanaged. However, it is also realized that each patient is different and so is each instance of the chronic condition being treated. As a result, symptom breakthrough and crises are likely to occur periodically over the period of treatment, which may demand reintervention or the design and implementation of entirely new packages of treatment. Throughout all of this management, the goal of the clinician, family members, and patient is to try to achieve an improvement in the quality of life and success for the individual who has ADHD.

References

•◆•

American Psychiatric Association. (1994). *Diagnostic and statistical manual of mental disorders* (4th ed.). Washington, DC: Author.

Barkley, R. A. (1995). *Taking charge of ADHD: The complete, authoritative guide for parents*. New York: Guilford Press.

Barkley, R. A. (1997a). Behavioral inhibition, sustained attention, and executive functions: Constructing a unifying theory of ADHD. *Psychological Bulletin, 121,* 65–94.

Barkley, R. A. (1997b). *ADHD and the nature of self-control*. New York: Guilford Press.

Barkley, R. A. (1998). *Attention-deficit/hyperactivity disorder: A handbook for diagnosis and treatment* (2nd ed.). New York: Guilford Press.

Bronowski, J. (1977). Human and animal languages. In *A sense of the future* (pp. 104–131). Cambridge, MA: MIT Press. (Reprinted from 1967, *To honor Roman Jakobson* [Vol. 1]. The Hague, Netherlands: Mouton)

Damasio, A. R. (1994). *Descartes' error: Emotion, reason, and the human brain.* New York: Putnam & Sons.

Damasio, A. R. (1995). On some functions of the human prefrontal cortex. In J. Grafman, K. J. Holyoak, & F. Boller (Eds.), Structure and functions of the human prefrontal cortex. *Annals of the New York Academy of Sciences, 769,* 241–251.

Ingersoll, P. D., & Goldstein, S. (1993). *Attention deficit disorder and learning disabilities: Realities, myths, and controversial treatments.* New York: Doubleday.

Werry, J., & Aman, M. (1999). *Practitioner's guide to psychoactive drugs for children and adolescents* (2nd ed.). New York: Plenum.

Suggested Reading

• ◆ •

The ADHD Report is a bimonthly newsletter for clinicians, edited by Dr. Barkley, with contributions from leading clinicians and researchers. Contact: Guilford Press (1-800-365-7006 or info@guilford.com)

Barkley, R. A. (1997). *ADHD and the nature of self-control.* New York: Guilford Press.

Barkley, R. A. (1997) *Defiant children* (2nd ed.): *A clinician's manual for assessment and parent training.* New York: Guilford Press.

Barkley, R. A. (1998). *Attention-deficit hyperactivity disorder: A handbook for diagnosis and treatment* (2nd ed.). New York: Guilford Press.

Barkley, R. A., & Benton, C. M. (1998). *Your defiant child: Eight steps to better behavior.* New York: Guilford Press.

Barkley, R. A., Edwards, G., & Robin, A. L. (1999). *Defiant teens: A clinician's manual for assessment and family intervention.* New York: Guilford Press.

Barkley, R. A., & Murphy, K. R. (1998). *Attention-deficit/hyperactivity disorder: A clinical workbook* (2nd ed.). New York: Guilford Press.

Children and Adults with Attention Deficit Disorder (CHADD). (1996). *ADD and adolescence: Strategies for success.* Landover, MD: Author.

DuPaul, G. J., Power, T. J., Anastopoulos, A. D., & Reid, R. (1998). *ADHD Rating Scale–IV: Checklists, norms, and clinical interpretation.* New York: Guilford Press.

DuPaul, G. J., & Stoner, G. (1994). *ADHD in the schools: Assessment and intervention strategies.* New York: Guilford Press.

Goldstein, S., & Goldstein, M. (1998). *Managing attention deficit hyperactivity disorder in children.* New York: Wiley.

Gordon, M., & McClure, D. (1997). *The down and dirty guide to adult ADHD.* DeWitt, NY: GSI.

Mash, E. J., & Barkley, R. A. (Eds.). (1996). *Child psychopathology.* New York: Guilford Press.

Mash, E. J., & Barkley, R. A. (Eds.). (1998). *Treatment of childhood disorders* (2nd ed.). New York: Guilford Press.

Nadeau, K. (1994). *A comprehensive handbook for attention deficit disorder in adults.* New York: Brunner/Mazel.

Parker, H. C. (1999). *Put yourself in their shoes: Understanding teenagers with attention-deficit hyperactivity disorder.* Plantation, FL: Specialty Press.

Robin, A. L. (1998). *ADHD in adolescents: Diagnosis and treatment.* New York: Guilford Press.

Weiss, G., & Hechtman, L. (1993). *Hyperactive children grown up* (2nd ed.). New York: Guilford Press.

Weiss, M., Hechtman, L., & Weiss, G. (1999). *ADHD in adulthood: A guide to current theory, diagnosis, and treatment.* Baltimore: Johns Hopkins University Press.

Wilens, T. E. (1999). *Straight talk about psychiatric medications for kids.* New York: Guilford Press.

Zentall, S. S., & Goldstein, S. (1999). *Seven steps to homework success.* Plantation, FL: Specialty Press.

Suggested Videos

•◆•

Barkley, R. A. (1993). *ADHD—What do we know?* New York: Guilford Press.

Barkley, R. A. (1993). *ADHD—What can we do?* New York: Guilford Press.

Barkley, R. A. (1994). *ADHD in adults.* New York: Guilford Press.

Barkley, R. A. (1994). *ADHD in the classroom: Strategies for teachers.* New York: Guilford Press.

Barkley, R. A. (1997). *Understanding the defiant child.* New York: Guilford Press.

Barkley, R. A. (1997). *Managing the defiant child.* New York: Guilford Press.

DuPaul, G. J., & Stoner, G. (1998). *Assessing ADHD in the schools.* New York: Guilford Press.

DuPaul, G. J., & Stoner, G. (1998). *Classroom interventions for ADHD.* New York: Guilford Press.

Resources

•◆•

The Attention Training System (ATS), an electronic token economy/response–cost system, is available from Gordon Systems, Inc., of DeWitt, New York. Gordon Systems maintains a website with information about ATS at www.gsi-add.com.

Additional training programs, assessment tools, educational games, books, videos, and newsletters are available from the ADD WareHouse of Plantation, Florida. The website address is www.addwarehouse.com.

About the Author

•◆•

Russell A. Barkley, PhD, is a professor of psychiatry and neurology at the University of Massachusetts Medical Center, Worcester, Massachusetts. He received his doctorate in 1977 in clinical psychology from Bowling Green State University in Ohio. He is a diplomate in both clinical psychology (ABPP) and clinical neuropsychology (ABCN, ABPP). Dr. Barkley has authored, coauthored, or coedited 14 books and clinical manuals. He has published more than 150 scientific articles and book chapters related to the nature, assessment, and treatment of ADHD. In 1993, he founded a bimonthly newsletter for clinical professionals, *The ADHD Report,* and currently serves as its editor. Dr. Barkley served as president of the Section of Clinical Child Psychology, Division 12, of the American Psychological Association, in 1988, and as president of the International Society for Research in Child and Adolescent Psychopathology in 1991. In 1994, he received the Distinguished Contribution Award from the American Association of Applied and Preventive Psychology. In 1996, he was awarded the C. Anderson Aldrich Award from the American Academy of Pediatrics for his research career in child development. Most recently (1998), he was awarded the Distinguished Contribution to Research Award from the Section of Clinical Child Psychology, Division 12, of the American Psychological Association.